CLASSICAL

MOXIBUSTION SKILLS

IN CONTEMPORARY

CLINICAL

PRACTICE

Sung Baek

BLUE POPPY PRESS ▪ 1990

BLUE POPPY PRESS

1775 Linden Avenue -- Boulder, CO 80304 -- (303) 442-0796

Edited and with a preface by James Ramholz, *L.Ac., Dipl.Ac. (NCCA)*. The editor wishes to acknowledge and thank Wilbur Rimes and Jerry Ostrowski for their invaluable help in preparing this monograph. This text originated from a postgraduate seminar -- Classical Moxibustion: History, Theory and Clinical Practice -- at the Chicago School of Oriental Medicine.

Distributors

AcuMedic CENTRE
101-105 CAMDEN HIGH STREET
LONDON NW1 7JN
Tel: 0171-388 5783/6704
Catalogue on Request

宋太醫竇材重集

扁鵲心書

通州張蹇署

Bian Que Xin Shu (Bian Que's Essential Writings), the title of the Song Dynasty text compiled by Dou Cai that Dr. Baek has primarily worked from in the preparation of this book. The overleaf is a reproduction of the title page from the original woodblock text.

PREFACE

Bian Que is one of the most famous physicians of Chinese antiquity. Known from the fifth or sixth century B.C., he is sometimes identified with Chun Yue-jen who is credited as being the first practitioner to write down the *Huang Di Ba Shi Yi Nan Jing*. He is traditionally considered a "holy" doctor who organized every part of Oriental medicine. Bian Que was the first specialist in moxibustion and founder of one of the two chief branches of moxibustion -- the other branch is named after Huang Di, the Yellow Emperor.

Moxibustion predates acupuncture. Instructions found in the book *Mencius* give a very early reference to the plant: "For any disease of seven years, seek three year old moxa." Although a much longer oral history is presumed, no therapeutic needling has been documented before 90 B.C. In 1973, a number of important documents were unearthed from the Ma Wang Tui graves which date back to 168 B.C. Interestingly enough, as well as containing medical texts which give us more information about the development and implementation of medical concepts, they also contained the oldest complete text of the *Dao De Jing*[1]. The medical texts predate both the *Shih-Chi* and the *Huang Di Nei Jing*. Paul Unschuld remarks that the medical texts from the Ma Wang Tui graves reveal that:

> Moxibustion, that is, the burning of powderized mugwort plants on the skin, is recommended as the *sole* stimulus for influencing the contents of the eleven vessels.[2] [Editor's emphasis]

Acupuncture was adopted and used to supplement moxa after the second century B.C. and a pharmacology of systematic correspondence was not developed until the early second century A.D.

During the Eastern Han Dynasty (c. 25 A.D. to 220 A.D.), moxa cones were moderately large and a considerable number were used. Later in the Tang (c. 618 A.D. to 907 A.D.) and Song (c. 960 A.D. to 1279 A.D.) Dynasties, up to one hundred cones were used. Indirect methods were developed and became widespread during the Tang and Qing Dynasties. Widely popular today is the method that originated during the Ming Dynasty of using a cigar-shaped roll. Herbs were also finely ground and added to the moxa roll to augment its therapeutic effect.

Taoist longevity methods recommend using large number of cones on particular points. One longevity method uses moxibustion on St.36 *(Zusanli)* -- one hundred cones if thirty years of age, two hundred cones if forty years old, etc. Another longevity method uses C.V.4 *(Guanyuan)* in the same way. Up to five hundred cones are used on C.V.4 *(Guanyuan)* after the

---

1. Ellen M. Chen, *The Tao Te Ching: A New Translation with Commentary*, Paragon House, New York, 1989, p.44

2. Paul U. Unschuld, *Medicine in China: A History of Ideas*, University of California Press, 1985, p.94

person is sixty years old. These types of treatments are done annually.

But this is not really medicine. The reason St.36 *(Zusanli)* is used is because it strengthens the digestive system so that the energy from the food can be utilized more efficiently, as well as helps supply the *Dan Tien*.

Current Moxibustion Practices

In the West, moxibustion has not enjoyed such widespread acceptance as acupuncture outside of the Chinese population. Textbooks devote little space to it and cauterization always presents the danger of scarring the patient if done improperly. Pictures of Chinese patients with moxa scars are not unfamiliar, but this form of blemish is unacceptable to most Western clients.

Contemporary opinion among practitioners considers this the most important prerequisite for moxibustion in the growing Western market -- that it not leave a scar.

> The new criterion distinguishes *only* whether or not cauterization leaves a scar.[3] [Editor's emphasis]

Moxibustion's importance in gerontology and difficult chronic problems, especially when complicated by deficiency, is highly undervalued and underutilized. It can be not only the most prudent but also the most effective way to treat severe problems. The foremost advantage of Bian Que moxa techniques is that despite the large number of cones used, virtually no scarring is done to the patient. Occasionally a small brown blemish which disappears in time is all that results from a treatment.

----

3. John O'Connor and Dan Bensky, Translators, *Acupuncture: A Comprehensive Text*, Eastland Press, Third Printing, 1984, p.400

While the typical TCM moxa therapies use large cones and provide a much broader application of heat to the acupuncture point and its surrounding area, the Japanese moxa therapies more closely resemble the classical Bian Que type of treatment. The moxa cones are very small threads or cones and the treatments plans are similar to Bian Que's. According to their styles, the patient often moxas every day at home for one month, increasing the number of cones weekly. Sometimes before an acupuncture treatment, a Japanese doctor will do direct moxa on T.W.4 *(Yangchi)* a few times with small cones to help build their weak patient's energy and help promote its circulation.

Selected Case Histories

Mr. R. W. Allopathic diagnosis: bronchial asthma. Pulse diagnosis showed deficient kidney energy. During the interview, the patient suffered a severe attack. His face turned pale with labored breathing. Three hundred moxa were burned on C.V.4 *(Guanyuan)*. After the twenty-fifth moxa, breathing became normal and facial color returned. After finishing the three hundred, the patient had no further attacks.

Mrs. A. in her middle 60's had failing eyesight. Fifty moxa were applied bilaterally to St.36 *(Zusanli)* once a month for three months. Deterioration of the vision stopped and eyesight improved.

Mr. C.J., age 59, a kidney dialysis patient had ankles swollen three times their natural size. Fifty moxa were applied bilaterally on Kd.1 *(Yongquan)*. Three hours after the treatment, the ankles were normal size.

Mr. J.M., age 72, had a lower back injury from a ladder fall during the winter. The injury was three years old and the patient suffered extreme lower back pain which was aggravated by cold and damp weather. The legs began to swell from the knee downward, and the patient complained of coldness throughout his body. Five hundred moxa were applied to C.V.4 *(Guanyuan)*. The pain disappeared, swelling cleared and the patient felt an overall increase of energy.

End Note

Sung Baek has an extensive background in acupuncture and herbalism. He currently teaches postgraduate acupuncture studies in Chicago, and is currently working on a new translation and commentary of the *Nei Jing*.

In this book, he has culled moxibustion formulas from a wide variety of traditional Korean, Japanese and Chinese sources as well as from his own clinical experience. Particularly noteworthy is *Bian Que's Essential Writings*, a book compiled during the Song Dynasty by the famous theoretician of that era Du Cai. Like other classics, it was probably a compilation of many authors' and editors' work over a number of years, which was then attributed to Bian Que.

Much of the best of what we know has already been with us a very long time. Like much of traditional Oriental medicine, moxibustion reached a level of sophistication a thousand years ago that has not been surpassed. With the production of this book, we hope it may be possible for contemporary practitioners to regain this expertise.

James Ramholz
Chicago,
November 1989

Table of Contents

CLASSICAL

THEORY

A cupuncture is a medicine of energy manipulation. Imagine the body as a series of reservoirs and locks filled with water. There might be an excess of pressure in one part and an absence in another. The differences in these pressures can be equalized *only* by draining the excess through the locks and bringing up the water level in the deficient reservoirs.

When you look at the imbalance, you must first stop the movement causing the abnormal pressures, and then decide through which channel the redistribution of pressure can be most efficiently accomplished. Abnormal movement of energy in the body distorts its balance, pulling and pushing in one part stronger than in another until a state of disease develops. Treatment aims at restoration of the original balance.

The techniques and methods applied during each session to restore this balance largely depend on the original cause of the disease and its level of development. The first thing to determine is whether the condition is an excess or a deficiency. If it is an excess, sedating or draining techniques are applied either by moving the energy to another part of the body where it can be utilized, or by completely draining it out of the body. If it is a

1

deficiency, we can tonify it by bringing the energy from a different area of the body or by adding new energy from outside the body.

The methods of treatment available include acupuncture, moxibustion, internal medicine, and other supplementary techniques, such as nutrition, exercise and physical therapy. And though the above methods often overlap, there are some general guidelines which should be followed in order to choose the best method. Since this book is limited to the discussion of moxibustion, we will concentrate on describing these areas where this type of therapy is most appropriate. And because it is often used as a complementary tool to acupuncture, I will try to clearly delineate the difference between these two methods.

Moxibustion can *add* new energy to the body. It can also be used when you discover points which are leaking energy out of the body. Moxa can be used for both excessive and deficient conditions. There are no contradictory circumstances to moxa -- proper selection of the acupuncture point for the treatment is the *only* thing that matters.

Some practitioners tend to associate moxibustion with deficiency points which are hollow, weak or concave. If they discover that type of point, they automatically think of applying moxibustion; but that is not the correct approach. If there is a certain organ, meridian or system of the body that has an excessive condition, you must drain that organ or meridian, and bring the energy to the deficient location through manipulation with needles.

As long as there is sufficient energy inside the body, you can manipulate that energy. If manipulation is not advisable because there is so much leakage that there is not enough energy to work with, then you must use moxa.

Moxibustion is preferable to herbal formulas because it is simpler, quicker and cheaper. It also manipulates energy much more directly. It's a direct route, unlike herbs which must move through the digestion and circulation systems first. For example, if a patient has a intestinal problem, but the stomach and spleen are also diseased, they will vomit the herbal formula. A second problem is that you do not have as precise control with herbs.

2

With moxibustion or acupuncture, you can constantly monitor the condition during treatment, as it changes through the pulse.

The general determination of how many times we moxa depends on the pulse. Typically, mild stimulation -- equivalent to using needles for tonification effect -- is three to seven cones. This method is the general rule when you moxa everyday. Classically, this was such a common presumption that few medical authors ever wrote it down: most sources just say moxa this point. The basic course for a moxibustion treatment is three to nine cones daily for four weeks; increasing the amount periodically, up to eleven cones. You can make the increase either weekly, biweekly or monthly.

In urgent cases when the patient is very deficient you must burn a lot at once -- up to fifty cones. For example, if there are severe stomach cramps due to cold energy and the back is sore, it means that the stomach has lost all of its yang energy. In such a case, you must use moxa if the other organs seem normal. Using acupuncture to change the balance would only weaken or endanger the other organs. In this case, you would moxa St.36 (*Zusanli*) or C.V.12 (*Zhongwan*) fifty times in a single treatment.

But it must be cautioned here that you can *not* substitute moxa for needles in an acupuncture formula. With moxa we can add energy and with needles we only manipulate the pre-existing energy of the system. Tonification by needling makes the energy flow stronger or supplies the energy from another part of the system. Sedation by needling stops the excessive or overactive energy flow in the meridian by slowing down or calming down the energy level. It does not remove energy from the system, but re-routes the energy flow to another channel. Through needling, we can control the relationship between two organs.

By actually taking energy out of the system, say through bleeding techniques, we may control the symptoms but may also break the balance with the other organs. In most cases, that energy does not have to be lost. You can view bleeding techniques as being diametrically opposite to moxa, because bleeding allows for energy to be released. The points you bleed are like valves which are opened to let pressure out of the system altogether.

Direct and Indirect Moxibustion

The terms "direct" and "indirect" moxibustion refers to how the moxa is applied. In the direct method, moxa is burned on the skin itself, sometimes utilizing a slice of an herb between the moxa and the skin. The primary benefit of direct moxa is its ability to add *new* energy -- that's why moxa has such a powerful effect on the body. You can put a touch of Vaseline or Arnica Ointment on the point before treatment to help the cones to stick upright and to help prevent burning.

Although indirect methods vary widely, the burning moxa never touches the skin. Therefore, larger quantities may be used and can supplement other therapies, such as needles or massage. The primary purpose of indirect moxa is to provide heat in order to "melt" something down -- this is a function of heat. For this purpose, any source of heat might do equally well. The heat harmonizes the energies in an area and provides yang energy support. This is needed in cases where the energy is frozen in certain areas. We must see that it is not deficient nor blocked, just frozen. You don't need to add any energy; just melt it with heat. That is easily done by indirect moxibustion.

For indirect moxa one uses a birdpecking technique which creates energy waves and pulses the heat into an area. However, when one does this, more than the acupuncture point is affected. The area is too large for the energy to become very concentrated. Moreover, neutralization of the moxa effect is possible by simultaneous stimulation of many unnecessary points close to it. When you do direct moxa on an acupuncture point correctly, the sensation is as if a thin needle has penetrated the skin very deep.

Moxibustion with Herbs

When we use direct moxa with herbs, it first of all lessens the chance of burning the skin. When you use slices of herbs under moxa, it diminishes the tonification function of the moxa but adds the energetic properties of the herb. Basically, you can pick any herb you wish as long as you use a thin slice.

When we use Aconite, it is for reinforcing strong yang energy. Garlic can be utilized for its effective detoxification properties. Ginger, being different from both aconite and garlic, is used for sedating superficial cold energy.

Indirect moxa, when used for skin disorders is herbal medicine, not strictly speaking moxibustion. When moxa is burned, it's smoke contains a chemical that has disinfectant properties. You could also wash the area with a decoction made from Artemesia to get the same effect. Sometimes it is necessary to burn moxa for skin problems but in such cases make sure that the smoke ends up touching the skin of the affected area. In order to make a wash instead, decoct the green rough type moxa wool in water, and rub the liquid onto the skin every three or four hours.

Making Moxa Cones

For direct moxibustion, the *smaller* the moxa cone, the better the tonification effect because you are not working with heat but with the energy. The *largest* moxa cone you should make for tonification is the size of a grain of rice. Cones larger than this will sedate the energy because the acupuncture points cannot handle that much energy at once.

For tonification the moxa should be very soft and light in color. The cones should be small and lightly packed. When you are ready to burn the moxa, place the cone lightly on the skin. Do not press it into the point, place it as if it was floating on the point, and burn an odd number of cones. Indirect moxa can also be burned on ginger, garlic or salt for tonification reasons.

You may also use moxa for sedation, or with sedation techniques. In these cases there is heat already present in the

5

system, and you don't want to loose it. For example, in the case of hot flashes due to deficient kidney energy, the organ is attempting to overcompensate for its low vitality and irregular function. Basically, heat is floating up because the organ producing the yang energy is weakened. This heat is false fire, and sedating it will further weaken an already deficient condition. Moxa should be used to pull the heat or floating yang energy back down to the lower warmer.

For sedation use the dark type of moxa. Make larger cones and press them tightly. When placing it on the skin press it into the point. When the moxa is burning blow it with your breath and let it burn faster. Burn even number of cones.

Course of Treatment

The normal course of treatment for moxibustion for the smaller formulas -- amounts of less than twenty cones -- is seven days a week for four weeks. In clinical practice, you may treat a patient for five days with two days rest; repeat this procedure for four weeks and then give a week's full rest. In the old Japanese moxibustion system, they often do this for three months. Then they would allow one full month of rest and then start the three month sequence again. This system is recommended for very chronic illness.

But in general, when you are working, for example on C.V.12 *(Zhongwan)* or St.36 *(Zusanli)* for digestive problems you can moxa each day for the entire month, or do it for five days with a two day break for four weeks. When we are doing these kinds of techniques, it may be necessary to let the patient do it at home, either by themselves or another family member.

Implementing the Treatment Plan

Indirect moxa is not a substitute for the direct method. If a patient cannot agree to undergo direct moxa in the office, the indirect method applied at home by the patient himself may prove fruitless or be impractical. The practitioner has less control over the circumstances, and the treatment may be less effective due to the patient's inconsistency.

Also there is no way to "double up" the treatments if the patient is not able to come each day. With moxa, it is very important that they get treated every day. You must follow the prescription's timetable. If you miss any treatment in the series, you must continue along the timetable as if it were not missed; you cannot increase dosage to catch up or make up the missing treatments.

So stick to the prescribed dosage. For example, three cones may be tonification, but four might already start to sedate the point. It's like a sine curve: as soon as the development reaches its limit it begins to reverse its effect. It all depends on the condition of the body and how the body responds to treatment. If you check the pulse and it shows significant improvement, you may not need to burn any more moxa because the condition could worsen by using more cones because of too forceful introduction of energy.

If after burning a few cones of moxa, the patient feels really comforted, that may be an indication that you have already burned enough cones. Check the pulse to verify the improvement. Moxibustion is like working on a wagon stuck on its way down a hill. Just give a push and it starts rolling. You don't have to help or push all the way down. The body will take care of the rest if all the other organs are not that disordered. If the body does not adjust itself, then you must start working on the other organs as well. But, to continue the analogy, you don't have to push the wagon all the way to the bottom.

When you moxa every day, gradually increase the dose. When starting the treatment, the patient will have the feeling of coolness and comfort with only a few burning. But after a while, that feeling will not be as clear with the same number of cones. Usually this takes place in about a week. It is at this time that you should increase the dosage by two cones. The standard texts in Chinese and Korean recommend increasing the moxibustion as the treatment progresses; but if the sensation of coolness and comfort lasts more than a week, then don't increase the number of cones. If the patient's condition has improved after one week, then you don't have to do any more to finish the course of the treatment.

The best time to stop moxibustion is when the patient tells you that it feels cool and comforting. The feeling of moxibustion should not be warming all over that area. They should feel like one sharp straight needle coming down, the deeper the better. And after that initial stimulation, they should feel the coolness. If you overdo moxibustion on a given area, one of the obvious signs that can occur is that the patient will begin swelling in that area.

TRADITIONAL

MOXIBUSTION

FORMULAS

Abdominal Pain

Due to Cold:
Moxa C.V.7 *(Yinjiao)*, twenty-one times.

Angina Pectoris

Special Point located one *cun* above C.V.15 *(Jiuwei)* on the sternum, one hundred times.

Arthritis

In general, moxa works much better than needles. But before moxa can be used, you have to be absolutely sure that there are no signs of inflammation. If there is any heat around the joints, needles should be used until all signs of heat are gone. Then the moxa treatment can begin. During the course of the treatment, attention should be paid to any signs of possible return of inflammation. If heat is observed, needles should be used again.

Whole Body:
Sp.6 *(Sanyinjiao)*
G.B.34 *(Yanglingquan)*
St.36 *(Zusanli)*
L.I.10 *(Shousanli)*
C.V.12 *(Zhongwan)*
G.B.18 *(Chengling)*
U.B.13 *(Feishu)*
Three to seven times each.

Spinal Arthritis:
Burn moxa between the vertebrae, three to seven times each.

Tuberculosis in all the joints:
U.B.13 *(Feishu)*
U.B.23 *(Shenshu)*
C.V.12 *(Zhongwan)*
L.I.11 *(Quchi)*
St.36 *(Zusanli)*
Sp.6 *(Sanyinjiao)*
Ahshi Points
Three to seven times each.

Knees:
Xiyan (Extra 32)
Three to seven times.

Asthma

1. Shortness of breath and asthma in old people:
C.V.4 *(Guanyuan)*, three hundred times.

2. When accompanied by lukewarm fever, bringing up blood from either the lung or stomach. The six pulses are wide, big, and tight when this condition is due to kidney energy damage: C.V.4 *(Guanyuan)*, three hundred times.

Bladder Problems

1. Incontinence:
C.V.4 *(Guanyuan)*, three hundred times.

2. Blood in urine -- especially when due to kidney energy damage from excessive sexual activity:
C.V.4 *(Guanyuan)*, four hundred times.

3. Infection -- especially due to kidney water damage:
C.V.4 *(Guanyuan)*, three hundred times.

Bleeding

1. Chronic vaginal or uterine bleeding:
C.V.3 *(Zhongji),* fourteen times.

2. Lower warmer or any area under the navel:
G.V.4 *(Mingmen)*, three to seven times.

3. General poor blood circulation:
St.36 *(Zusanli)*, seven to eleven times.

Body Odor

For repulsive armpit odor:
Moxa Ht.1 *(Jiquan)*, ten times.

Chronic Diseases

To tonify the general vitality and triple warmer energy before needling:
Moxa T.W.4 *(Yangchi)*, three to seven times.

Colitis

1. When perverse energy attacks through the anus:
Moxa Lu.6 *(Kongzui)*, three to seven times.

2. Extra Point 2 *cun* below Lu.6 *(Kongzui)*, three to seven times.

Constipation

1. C.V.7 *(Yinjiao)*, three times.

2. Ht.7 *(Shenmen)*, three times.

3. In older patients who are weak or weakened by prolonged illness, especially when they cannot take tonification herbs:
C.V.8 *(Shenque)*, one hundred times.

Death Pulse

C.V.4 *(Guanyuan)*, five hundred times.

Diarrhea

General diarrhea: moxa Pc.8 *(Laogong)* three to five times.

Morning diarrhea: moxa U.B.60 *(Kunlun)* twenty to thirty times.

If accidently caused by moxa treatment of L.I.11 *(Quchi)*:
Sedate G.V.26 *(Renzhong)*.

Diabetes

Due to heart and kidney damaged by heat and the patient is
extremely thirsty and drinks a great amount of water; or when
cold energy damages the lung and kidney:

C.V.4 *(Guanyuan)*, one hundred times, or
C.V.6 *(Qihai)*, one hundred times.

We use C.V.6 in the spring because energy is growing and the
kidney energy is already at its peak; so we can work in a higher
part of the body. In this case even if we use C.V.6, we are still
tonifying C.V.4. and the *Dan Tien.*

Dizziness

This treatment will strengthen the liver and gall bladder for
women exposed to wind, without any other symptoms:
Moxa C.V.12 *(Zhongwan)*, fifty times.

Edema

1. Chest area type caused by lung energy:
Lu.2 *(Yumen)*, one hundred times.

2. Whole body type:
C.V.4 *(Guanyuan)*, five hundred times.

3. Due to extreme spleen damage; especially when showing
urinary retention or inability to breath when lying down:
Sp.17 *(Shidou)*, two hundred times and
C.V.4 *(Guanyuan)*, three hundred times.

Emergency

C.V.8 *(Shenque)*, one hundred times.

Eyes, Ears, Nose, Throat and Mouth

Ears -- Middle ear infection:
A.
T.W.17 *(Yifeng)*
T.W.21 *(Ermen)*
S.I.19 *(Tinggong)*
Each three times.

B.
T.W.17 *(Yifeng)*
G.B.2 *(Tinghui)*
L.I.10 *(Shousanli)*
L.I.4 *(Hegu)*
Kd.6 *(Zhaohai)*
Each five to seven times.

Eyes
1. Myopia:
A.
L.I.19 *(Heliao)*
Lv.8 *(Ququan)*
U.B.23 *(Shenshu)*
C.V.12 *(Zhongwan)*
U.B.10 *(Tianzhu)*
G.B.34 *(Yanglingquan)*
Each three to seven times.

2. Night blindness:
Use a Special Point located on the biggest wrinkle of the first
joint of the yang side of the thumb, five to seven times.

3. Cataract due to exhaustion of spleen and kidney:

C.V.4 *(Guanyuan)*, three hundred times.

Nose
1. Polyps:
G.V.23 *(Shangxing)*
One to fifteen times after needling to a depth of one-fifth to one-fourth inch.

2. Loss of sense of smell:
L.I.20 *(Yingxiang)*, three to seven times with very small cones.

3. Epistaxsis:
Special Point located one-half below G.V.15 *(Yamen)*, three times.

Sore throat
1. L.I.4 *(Hegu)*, three to seven times.

2. Lu.8 *(Jingqu)*, three times.
Important: use very small cones, and never moxa more than three times or you could injure the general vitality.

3. Tip of the medial malleolus seven times. If it does not work, also moxa the lateral side.

4. Chronic sore throat and loss of voice:
C.V.4 *(Guanyuan)*, three hundred times.

Toothache:
A. Special Point located on the back side of the first joint of the middle finger, moxa seven times.

B. Special Point located in the anatomical snuff box, seven times.

Facial Palsy

1. General
A.
L.I.4 *(Hegu)*, seven to nine times on both sides.

B.
G.V.21 *(Qianding)*
L.I.11 *(Quchi)*
St.36 *(Zusanli)*
G.V.17 *(Naohu)*

C. St.4 *(Dicang)*
Thirty times. If wind enters through the ears causing paralysis, moxa twenty-seven to fifty times.

2. Chronic:
St.36 *(Zusanli)*
St.4 *(Dicang)*
U.B.18 *(Ganshu)*
Moxa each daily seven times on both sides. This treatment may take many months.

Fever

L.I.11 *(Quchi)*, fourteen times.

Gall Stones

G.B.24 *(Riyue)*, seven to nine times.

Gonorrhea

A. General
1. Moxa G.V.1 *(Changqiang)* twenty times each day for seven days.

2.
C.V.6 *(Qihai)*
U.B.25 *(Dachangshu)*
U.B.28 *(Pangguangshu)*
C.V.3 *(Zhongji)*
C.V.2 *(Qugu)*
St.36 *(Zusanli)*
Sp.6 *(Sanyinjiao)*
S.I.5 *(Yanggu)*
Each five to seven times.

3.
U.B.27 *(Xiaochangshu)*
U.B.22 *(Sanjiaoshu)*
C.V.5 *(Shimen)*
C.V.6 *(Qihai)*
Sp.2 *(Dadu)*
Moxa three to five times.

B. Gonorrhea accompanied by bleeding:
1. Moxa G.V.4 *(Mingmen)*, fifty to seventy times.
2. Moxa Sp.6 *(Sanyinjiao)*, and C.V.2 *(Qugu)* nine times.

Head Pain

General type:
U.B.7 *(Tongtian)*, seven times for seven days.

Lateral type:
Lu.10 *(Yuji)*, opposite side of pain, five times.

Migraine:
G.B.18 *(Chengling)*, twenty-one times.

Heat Separation

Kd.1 *(Yongquan)*, seven to eleven times.

Hepatitis

Yin type:
C.V.4 *(Guanyuan)*, three hundred times.

Hemiplegia

1. L.I.11 *(Quchi)*, fourteen times.

2. Due to exogenous wind and damp entering into the organs. Or when the two eyeballs move separately and both hands are very stiff. Both of these are traditionally called false *Zhong Feng*. Moxa the back *Shu* points belonging to the yin organs.

A.
U.B.13 *(Feishu)*, fifty times.

B.
U.B.13 *(Feishu)*
U.B.15 *(Xinshu)*
Each fifty times.

C.
U.B.18 *(Ganshu)*
U.B.23 *(Shenshu)*
Each fifty times.

D.
U.B.13 *(Feishu)*
U.B.15 *(Xinshu)*
U.B.18 *(Ganshu)*
U.B.20 *(Pishu)*

U.B.23 *(Shenshu)*
Moxa each fifty times.

Hernia

General
1. First you must find the Special Point by measuring the distance between the two St.4 *(Dicang)* points with a string. Then form an equilateral triangle, each side of which is one-third the distance between the two point. The first upper angle of the triangle is formed by the navel, the two lower angles are the points we are looking for.

2. Moxa C.V.4 *(Guanyuan)*, one hundred times.

A.
Herniated intestines:
C.V.4 *(Guanyuan)*, nine to fifty times.

B.
First you must find a special point. Measure the distance between the two St.4 *(Dicang)* points with a string. Then form an equilateral triangle, each side of which is one-third the distance between the two point. The first upper angle of the triangle is formed by the navel, the two lower angles are the points we are looking for.

Herpes

1. G.V.4 *(Mingmen)*, thirty times.

2.
U.B.22 *(Sanjiaoshu)*
C.V.5 *(Shimen)*
Each twenty times.

3.
C.V.5 *(Shimen)*
C.V.6 *(Qihai)*
Moxa three to five times each.

4.
U.B.27 *(Xiaochangshu)*
U.B.22 *(Sanjiaoshu)*
C.V.5 *(Shimen)*
C.V.6 *(Qihai)*
Moxa three to five times.

High Blood Pressure

Kd.1 *(Yongquan)*, ten to twenty times with larger cones.

Impotence and Fertility

1. Men's sexual deficiency:

A. C.V.3 *(Zhongji)*, ten to thirty times.

B. U.B.22 *(Sanjiaoshu)*, ten to thirty times.

C. Lv.1 *(Dadun)*, five to seven times.

D. Moxa both C.V.4 *(Guanyuan)* and C.V.3 *(Zhongji)* three times the first week, five times the second week, seven times the third week, and nine times the fourth week.

E. Sp.1 *(Yinbai)*, three to seven times.

F. *Huatuo* points of the lower thoracic and the lumbar region, each three times daily.

G. C.V.4 *(Guanyuan)*, three hundred times. Especially useful for extreme exhaustion and lack of erection or spermatogenic problem in the male.

2. Women's sexual deficiency and infertility:

A. Kd.13 *(Qixue)*, five to fifty times.

B. Frequent miscarriage:
Lv.11 *(Yinlian)*, ten to twenty times.

C. Lack of sex drive and lubrication:
C.V.4 *(Guanyuan)*, three hundred times.

Indigestion

Overeating or when the food itself is the cause of stagnation:
Lu.1 *(Zhongfu)*, fifty times.

Infection

A. Reproductive organs, bladder or kidney:
Lu.7 *(Lieque)*, fifty times.

B. Intestines:
L.I.10 *(Shousanli)*, one hundred times.

Insanity and Other Mental Disorders

1. Insanity
A. Lu.11 *(Shaoshang)*, five to seven times or until the patient feels hot on the finger.

B. For haunted or psychiatric patients:
Ghost Crying Points, seven times.

This point is found at the same level and lateral to Lu.11 *(Shaoshang)*. Place the patient's palms together and tie with thread. Where the thumbs touch, burn both points at the same time with a single cone.

C. Special Point located between the spinous process of the second and third thoracic vertebrae.

D.
C.V.12 *(Zhongwan)*
C.V.4 *(Guanyuan)*
Moxa each three hundred times.

E. Lu.9 *(Taiyuan)*, seven times.

2. Ghost possession:
Ghost possession in terms of Oriental medicine means that their heart, liver and mind are weak and they are easily manipulated by their environment and external influences.

A. C.V.14 *(Juque)* fifty times, and C.V.4. *(Guanyuan)*, three hundred times.

B. Especially when confused, looses awareness and personality:
G.B.21 *(Jianjing)*, fifty times.

3. Depression:
Lv.3 *(Taichong)*, thirty times, especially if caused by liver deficiency or point shows pain.

Jaundice

A. Yellow or black:
Sp.17 *(Shidou)*, two hundred times.

B. When accompanied by pus on the neck or spine, or any toxicity of the skin:
C.V.4 *(Guanyuan)*, three hundred times.

Joint Pain, Weakness or Numbness

1. Finger Spasm:
Five Tiger Points *(Wuhu*, M-UE-45), three to seven times.

2. Wrist: Lu.7 *(Liehque)*, seven times.

3. Weakness of Arm with Pain in Elbow or Shoulder:
L.I.11 *(Quchi)*, fourteen times.

4. Shoulder:
A. L.I.14 *(Binao)*, three to seven times.

B. L.I.15 *(Jianyu)*, three to seven times.

C. S.I.10 *(Naoshu)*, three to seven times.

D. T.W.14 *(Jianliao)*, three to seven times.

5. Knee:
A. St.35 *(Dubi)*, three to seven times.

B. St.36 *(Zusanli)*, three to seven times for knee and leg disorders.

C. Moxa *Ahshi* points.

6. Leg:
A. Kd.1 *(Yongquan)*, fifty times.

B. Stiffness through the legs and lower back, especially when due to loss of kidney energy through excessive sexual activity:

C.V.4 *(Guanyuan)*, five hundred times.

7. Lumbar and sacrum:
A. U.B.22 *(Sanjiaoshu)* can be used along with U.B.23 *(Shenshu)* and U.B.25 *(Dachangshu)* for all kinds of lumbar and kidney problems including sciatica, low back pain, and sexual energy weakness. Moxa here daily three times during the first week, five times during the second week, seven times during the third week, and nine the fourth week.

B. Kidney deficiency type:
1.
St.36 *(Zusanli)*
U.B.22 *(Sanjiaoshu)*
U.B.25 *(Dachangshu)*
Each three to seven times.

2.
U.B.22 *(Sanjiaoshu)*
U.B.23 *(Shenshu)*
U.B.25 *(Dachangshu)*
especially when accompanied by impotence, three to seven times.

C. Due to cold and damp energy:
G.V.2 *(Yaoshu)*, fifty times.

Kidney Damage

1. Both ears show dryness and grayish or black color:
C.V.4 *(Guanyuan)*, five hundred times.

2. Patients over forty years of age with dry mouth and tongue, without salivation because kidney is not generating water energy:
C.V.4 *(Guanyuan)*, three hundred times.

3. Patients over forty years of age with strong pain in the lower back and sacrum area:
C.V.4 *(Guanyuan)*, three hundred times.

4. Inflammation of the skin of the groin area. The kidney energy is being attacked by perverse wind and it is penetrating to the bone. This condition can threaten future bone disease:
C.V.4 *(Guanyuan)*, two hundred times.

5. Older patients whose breathing is short and shallow because the kidney energy is not returning from the lung to the kidney. In other words, the connection between the lung and kidney is cut. In this case, patients may be hyperventilating:
C.V.4 *(Guanyuan)*, two hundred times.

Labor and Delivery

1. Strengthen uterus before delivery:
C.V.6 *(Qihai)*, several days before delivery, nine to fifteen times.

2. Fetus is dead but will not come out:
C.V.3 *(Zhongji)*, fifty-three times.

3. To increase general vitality after delivery:
L.I.4 *(Hegu)*, fifty to one hundred times.

4. Anemia after delivery:
C.V.12 *(Zhongwan)*, four hundred times.

Liver Disorders

General:
C.V.12 *(Zhongwan)*

Lv.14 *(Qimen)* on the right side
U.B.18 *(Ganshu)*
U.B.19 *(Danshu)*
U.B.23 *(Shenshu)*
G.B.34 *(Yanglingquan)*
Sp.6 *(Sanyinjiao)*
Moxa each five to seven times.

Edema caused by the liver:
1. C.V.9 *(Shuifen)*, five to twenty times.

2. Special point located one and one-half *cun* lateral to C.V.9 *(Shuifen)*.

Infection of the liver:
U.B.19 *(Danshu)*
St.40 *(Fenglong)*
C.V.12 *(Zhongwan)*
L.I.11 *(Quchi)*
St.36 *(Zusanli)*
Lv.14 *(Qimen)*
Sp.6 *(Sanyinjiao)*
G.B.20 *(Fengchi)*
Moxa each five to seven times.

Longevity and Prevention of Disease

1. L.I.14 *(Binao)*, seven times.

2. Moxa C.V.4 *(Guanyuan)* according to age:
A. If in the 30s, thirty-five times every three years.

B. If in the 50s, one hundred times every two years.

C. If in the 60s, three hundred times annually.

3. St.36 *(Zusanli)*, fifty times for prevention of disease and general health maintenance by tonifying the yin energy.

Lung Problems

Huatuo Points next to the 7, 8, 9, 10, and 11TH thoracic vertebrae.

Malaria

1. G.V.14 *(Dazhui)*, sixty times.

2. Malaria caused by spleen deficiency or damage. This treatment helps relieve fever and chill symptoms by helping the earth element:
A. Sp.17 *(Shidou)*, five hundred times. Especially when the immune system is down.

B. C.V.12 *(Zhongwan)* one hundred times and Sp.17 *(Shidou)* on the left side one hundred times.

Menstrual Disorders

1. Irregular:
C.V.3 *(Zhongji)*, three times daily.

2. Uterine spasm:
C.V.4 *(Guanyuan)*, twenty-one times.

3. Menopause:
C.V.4 *(Guanyuan)*, thirty times.

4. Delayed or Lack:
Kd.13 *(Qixue)*, five to fifty times; often ten times is enough.

Osteoporosis

C.V.4 *(Guanyuan)*, three hundred times.

Paralysis

1. One-sided, with loss of voice and kidney deficiency:
Moxa C.V.4 *(Guanyuan)* five hundred times. If the stroke occurs because of nerve or kidney damage, this is an ideal formula. But if the origin is due to diabetes, spleen damage, or heat ascending then this method will not work as well, although it will strengthen such patients during the course of treatment.

2. Mild paralysis with little or no sensation or difficulty in movement:
G.V.20 *(Baihui)*, thirty times
G.B.21 *(Jianjing)*, fifty times
L.I.11 *(Quchi)*, fifty times
St.36 *(Zusanli)*, fifty times.
Moxa all points in a single treatment.

Pneumonia, Common Cold, Flu and Coughing

1. Locate the Special Point located three *cuns* lateral to the nipple and moxa it three to seven times. In the male use the left side, in the female the right.

2. Lung damage due to cold energy or when coughing continues after the original problem is gone, especially in patients over forty years of age:
C.V.4 *(Guanyuan)*, three hundred times.

3. Chronic coughing due to cold stagnating in the lung:
C.V.22 *(Tientu)*, fifty times.

4. Chronic cough:
U.B.17 *(Geshu)*, fifty times.

Sciatica

1.
U.B.22 *(Sanjiaoshu)*
U.B.23 *(Shenshu)*
U.B.25 *(Dachangshu)*

2.
U.B.22 *(Sanjiaoshu)*
U.B.23 *(Shenshu)*
U.B.25 *(Dachangshu)*
U.B.37 *(Yinmen)*
U.B.60 *(Kunlun)*
G.B.34 *(Yanglingquan)*
St.36 *(Zusanli)*
Moxa each three times.

3. G.V.2 *(Yaoshu)*, thirty times.

4. C.V.4 *(Guanyuan)*, fifty to one hundred times.

Seizures

1. G.V.20 *(Baihui)* and G.V.23 *(Shangxing)*, seven times.

2. G.V.20 *(Baihui)*, seven times.

3. G.V.20 *(Baihui)*, seven times.

4. C.V.24 *(Chengjiang)*, one hundred times.

5. C.V.12 *(Zhongwan)*, four hundred times for epileptic-type seizure with fainting and convulsions or trembling.

Shang Han

Shao Yin condition:
The patient's six pulses are floating. They display great confusion and speak without consciousness. Their body feels heavy to them and exhibits a grayish black complexion, swelling of the stomach, vomiting with mucus, and toes are cold:
Moxa C.V.4 *(Guanyuan)*, five hundred times.

Tai Yin condition:
Body and legs are cold. The six pulses are tight and big. Yellowish coloring with purplish spots on the skin. Dry vomiting. High fever with lack of salivation. Dizziness.
Moxa C.V.12 *(Zhongwan)*, one hundred times

Skin Infection

1. Local Area:
Bleed randomly with a spring needle, and then use moxa smoke or make a decoction and soak repeatedly.

A. Back of the hand, L.I.11 *(Quchi)*, fifty times.

B. Pus on skin around G.V.26 *(Renzhong)* point:
C.V.5 *(Shimen)*, one hundred times.

2. Whole body:
Zhuchun (at the tip of the olecranon), seven times.

C. Allergy:
Sp.10 *(Xuehai)*, five to seven times for five to seven days.

D. Perverse wind and damp disturbing the inner organs:
U.B.13 *(Feishu)*
U.B.23 *(Shenshu)*
U.B.15 *(Xinshu)*

U.B.20 *(Pishu)*
U.B.18 *(Ganshu)*

E. Dryness and psoriasis
Do moxibustion three *cun* away from the center of the dry patch. Usually, if you can pick out the meridian direction, choose two points, one above and below. But if the meridian line is not clear, pick out four points -- one at each corner. If the points secrete a yellow liquid (which is usually lymph), then it is a sign of healing. Continue this treatment until the liquid does come.

Sore Throat

1. L.I.4 *(Hegu)*, three to seven times.

Speech Problems

A. Accompanied by shortness of breath:
Moxa Lu.5 *(Chize)*, one hundred times.

B. For paralysis patients when the kidney and lung energies are damaged:
C.V.4 *(Guanyuan)*, five hundred times.

Spleen Related Problems

1. Bian Que's method for all types of spleen related problems typically includes the use of Sp.17 *(Shidou)*.

A. For any excessive or deficient problem of the spleen itself:
Moxa Sp.17 *(Shidou)* five hundred times.

B. Damage to the spleen, stomach and kidney organs in summer showing dry heat because of excessive consumption

of cold food. Avoid giving cold herbs because they will cut the energy connection between the three warmers *(San Jiao)*:
Sp.17 *(Shidou)*, one hundred times.

2. If the patient shows strong pain in the middle of the chest or around the diaphragm:
Sp.17 *(Shidou)*, fifty times.

3. Spleen damage showing black or yellowish color on the face and loss of appetite:
Sp.17 *(Shidou)*, fifty times. If the patient has pale facial coloring due to kidney damage, moxa C.V.4 *(Guanyuan)* two hundred times also.

Stagnation Symptoms

1. Intestinal swelling caused by blood or water stagnation:
L.I.10 *(Shousanli)*, one hundred times.

2. Chest congestion with burning sensation:
L.I.11 *(Quchi)*, fourteen times.

3. Chest area:
C.V.5 *(Shimen)*, one hundred times.

4. Lower abdomen:
C.V.6 *(Qihai)*, one hundred times.

E. Cold hands and feet:
Sp.2 *(Dadu)*, one hundred times.

F. Energy blockage causing cramps or spasm of stomach:
C.V.12 *(Zhongwan)*, five hundred times.

Stomach and Digestion Problems

A. Cross Formula:
Tonification of the appetite and most stomach disorders. It can be used for cancer, tumor, chronic indigestion, ulcers, spasm of the stomach, etc. It can also be used for related hepatitis and gall stones.
C.V.11 *(Jianli)*
C.V.12 *(Zhongwan)*
C.V.13 *(Shangwan)*
St.21 *(Liangmen)*

B. Acute Stomach Pain:
C.V.12 *(Zhongwan)*, ten times.

C. Spasms:
1. St.21 *(Liangmen)*, until spasms stop.

2. *Jungchoo* (the Korean name of a special point located below the 10TH thoracic vertebrae), thirty times.

D. Chronic digestive organ disease:
Huatuo Points next to thoracic 7, 8, 9, 10, & 11, fifteen to twenty times.

Sweating

1. When patient cannot sweat:
Moxa Lu.6 *(Kongzui)*, fifty times

Throat Problems

When Inflammation, swelling or constriction of the throat create an inability to swallow:
C.V.22 *(Tiantu)*, fifty times.

Toothache

Lu.7 *(Lieque)*, seven times.

Urination Problems

Moxa C.V.9 *(Shuifen)* three times per treatment the first week, five times the second, seven times the third, and eleven times on the fourth week.

Vomiting

1. Lu.5 *(Chize)*, three to seven times.

2. Due to cold energy damage to the stomach:
C.V.12 *(Zhongwan)*, fifty times.

If this patient shows cold legs and arms and the six pulses are thin, moxa C.V.4 *(Guanyuan)* three hundred times to save the yang energy.

Zhong Feng

1. Kd.1 *(Yongquan)* and G.V.14 *(Dazhui)* thirty times.

2. Partial paralysis without stroke:
C.V.12 *(Zhongwan)*, four hundred times.
Paralysis may be either on the left or right side. The left side indicates a stomach problem; the right side, a liver or gall bladder problem.

ADVANCED

MOXIBUSTION

SKILLS

T he formulations given below are designed for extremely serious or urgent problems caused by the deficiency of the related organ. The patient's own energy is so low that there is not enough available for effective acupuncture manipulation.

These moxa formulas are meant to be performed in a *single* treatment. The practitioner should continuously monitor the changes in the pulse; often fewer cones than prescribed will give the desirable result.

The practitioner will notice that the same prescription is often recommended for a variety of problems. Since it is the belief of the translator that the originators of these moxa formulas repeated them in order to underscore their importance, we have decided to follow the original outline as much as possible.

1. For all general male and female physical exhaustion. In men's cases, including impotence -- both the lack of erection and spermatogenesis. In women, if they don't have any drive or vaginal lubrication:

C.V.4 *(Guanyuan)*, three hundred times.

2. For osteoporosis or yin-type hepatitis:

C.V.4 *(Guanyuan)*, three hundred times.

3. Lung damage caused by common cold or flu. The patient keeps on coughing after the original cold is gone:

C.V.4 *(Guanyuan)*, three hundred times.

4. For chronic sore throat, or if they keep on loosing their voice:

C.V.4 *(Guanyuan)*, three hundred times.

5. Shortness of breath or asthma in old persons:

C.V.4 *(Guanyuan)*, three hundred times.

6. Chronic and acute seizures. This includes epilepsy or any case where a patient loses consciousness with convulsions:

C.V.12 *(Zhongwan)*, four hundred times.

7. Anemia after delivery, or women who are chronically anemic and have heavy periods:

C.V.12 *(Zhongwan)*, fifty times.

8. Partial paralysis, chronic or acute, *not* caused by stroke. Either on the left or the right side of the body. Left side indicates a

stomach problem; right side indicates a liver or gall bladder problem:

C.V.12 *(Zhongwan)*, four hundred times.

9. For ghost possession -- which means that the patient's heart, liver and mind are weak and that they can be easily manipulated by the external environment. External stimulation, visual, sound, etc. easily changes them. If you see this kind of case you can treat them as a ghost possession:

C.V.14 *(Juque)*, fifty times
C.V.4 *(Guanyuan)*, three hundred times.

10. Dizziness in women when they are exposed to wind without any other obvious cause:

C.V.12 *(Zhongwan)*, fifty times.

11. Ghost possession or a mental condition in which a patient becomes confused and looses personality and awareness:

G.V.21 *(Jianjing)*, fifty times.

12. In case of death pulse, immediately moxa:

C.V.4 *(Guanyuan)*, five hundred times.

13. For water retention causing whole body edema:

C.V.4 *(Guanyuan)*, five hundred times.

14. For chronic malaria caused by spleen deficiency. In this case the immune system is not functioning. This formula helps the hot and cold energy balance by strengthening the spleen:

Sp.17 *(Shidou)*, five hundred times.

15. In cases where the energy flow is blocked causing wild energy behavior in certain parts of the body. For instance, an energy block around the stomach can cause problems elsewhere, such as cramps:

C.V.12 *(Zhongwan)*, five hundred times.

16. Yellow or black jaundice:
Sp.17 *(Shidou)*, two hundred times.

17. Any spleen problem -- it can be excessive or deficient:

Sp.17 *(Shidou)*, five hundred times.

18. Elderly patient's bladder-control problems:

C.V.4 *(Guanyuan)*, three hundred times.

19. Neuralgia-type pain accompanied by swollen and weak leg:

Kd.1 *(Yongquan)*, fifty times.

20. Summertime stomach pain, accompanied by stomach spasms. It is caused by cold energy inside when people over-cool themselves in the summer:

C.V.4 *(Guanyuan)*, thirty times.

21. Exhaustion in women during delivery causing edema:

C.V.4 *(Guanyuan)*, three hundred times.

22. Edema after delivery:

C.V.4 *(Guanyuan)*, three hundred times
Sp.17 *(Shidou)*, one hundred times.

23. Kidney energy deficiency causing the face or body color to turn gray or blackish:

C.V.4 *(Guanyuan)*, five hundred times.

24. Continuous vomiting with inability to eat:

C.V.12 *(Zhongwan)*, fifty times.

ESSENTIAL

MOXIBUSTION

POINTS

Sp.17 *(Shidou)*

Bian Que called this point *Mingguan* or life gate. It is directly connected to the true energy of the spleen. By manipulating this point we directly manipulate the energy of the spleen. This point controls all spleen related diseases. If there is at least a bit of energy left in the spleen it is advisable to moxa Sp.17 *(Shidou)* two hundred to three hundred times; this way we revive the spleen energy and keep the patient from spleen death.

Use this point for all serious diseases based on a spleen problem. Helping the spleen means helping the mother of all five organs. The spleen is the organ responsible for the creation of vital energy of the body. It is the organ creating the vital energy, other then the energy we are born with. The spleen grows and nourishes the other organs. All the nourishing energy for the organs resides in the spleen. One should moxa Sp.17 *(Shidou)* for an illness with various symptoms that don't heal. Great results can often seen.

Spleen emergencies can include severe indigestion, inability of the body to control the water metabolism, and rheumatic heart disease.

U.B.23 *(Shenshu)*

For all general serious weakness, moxa U.B.23 *(Shenshu)* two hundred to three hundred times. This point tonifies the kidney, and tonificaton of the kidney means nourishing the root of the whole body. Kidney energy is the vital energy. If the kidney energy is very strong, the patient will not die. Use U.B.23 *(Shenshu)* for paralysis, loss of voice, numbness of the limbs and an illness accompanied by seizures.

U.B.57 *(Chengshan)*

This point is used for beriberi. When the legs are heavy, the patient cannot walk and shows painful swelling, moxa this point fifty to one hundred times.

G.V.2 *(Yaoshu)*

For lower backache and for women whose sacral area is very painful after delivery or for lumbosacral arthritis, moxa fifty times.

Kd.1 *(Yongquan)*

This point is good for sore legs, beriberi, when the center of the foot is painful, when the big toe or side of the foot is painful -- basically for most foot and sole problems.

You can burn moxa in two different ways at this point in order to warm the middle warmer: use larger moxa cones to sedate the cold and bring down the heat; or use small moxa cones in order to slowly add heat, building it up from the bottom.

St.36 *(Zusanli)*

Locate this point with the knees flexed. It is used for patients who start loosing their eyesight. It is also good for swollen, painful, and heavy knee joints; especially when the patient shows difficulty in walking.

If by mistake you give too much heat through C.V.12 *(Zhongwan)* or C.V.4 *(Guanyuan)* the patient will develop dermatitis. If you moxa St.36 *(Zusanli)* the heat will go down.

You can use both Kd.1 *(Yongquan)* or St.36 *(Zusanli)* to bring the heat down. If the heat is in the top area use Kd.1 *(Yongquan)*; if it is on the surface use St.36 *(Zusanli)*.

G.B.18 *(Chengling)*

This is a very important point for migraines. Burn moxa here twenty-one times. Burning moxa cones here usually provides very good results.

G.B.15 *(Linqi)*

For migraine headache with *Tai Yang* energy, or what in Oriental medicine is actually called a "brainache". Moxa this point forty times.

Tianding (A Special Point, not L.I.17)

At the time when *Bian Que's Essential Writings* was compiled, *Tianding* was the name for a point located three and one-half *cuns* above U.B.3 *(Meichong)*. This point can be used for pain on the top of the head, especially when the patient is loosing eyesight at the same time.

EMERGENCY

TECHNIQUES

In this section, when two points are burned in one formula it usually means that there is an involvement of two organs. The practitioner must decide which organ is in more urgent circumstances and moxa it first. But once that organ builds up sufficient energy, both points can be done at once.

1. One-sided paralysis, loss of voice, accompanied by kidney deficiency:

C.V.4 *(Guanyuan)*, five hundred times

2. *Shao Yin* condition of *Shang Han*
The patient's six pulses are floating, and there is great confusion and speech without consciousness. The body feels heavy and there is grayish black complexion. There is swelling of the stomach and vomiting of mucous. The toes are cold.

C.V.4 *(Guanyuan)*, three hundred times.

3. *Tai Yin* condition of *Shang Han*

The six pulses are tight and big. The body and legs are cold, with yellowish color and purplish spots on the skin. There is dry vomit with high fever, lack of salivation and dizziness.

C.V.4 *(Guanyuan)*, three hundred times
Sp.17 *(Shidou)*, three hundred times.

The above two are the most dangerous conditions of *Shang Han*. They can destroy the health extremely fast. Dryness of the mouth and tongue are characteristic signs of the *Shao Yin* stage; whereas abdominal distention and diarrhea are characteristic of the *Tai Yin* stage.

Tonifying the kidney here does not give heat to the *Shao Yin* condition. Rather, it is essentially strengthening the kidney. So using other remedies to increase the heat in the body is not allowed because they will only promote the rising of heat. Moxibustion on C.V.4 *(Guanyuan)* increases the *Yuan Qi* of the kidney, thus promoting the vital energy to fight any pathogenic factors.

4. Jaundice accompanied by pus on the neck and spine, or any toxicity of the skin, is also a very urgent case. Pus on head and the cervical area are considered very serious because it can attack the central nervous system. In these situations, we have to tonify the kidney energy.

C.V.4 *(Guanyuan)*, three hundred times.

5. Acute inflammation of the throat or constriction of the throat with swelling causing an inability to swallow food when caused by deficiency of the stomach meridian or wind and cold attacking the lung.

C.V.22 *(Tiantu)*, fifty times.

6. Pneumonia or asthma accompanied by lukewarm fever, vomiting of blood either from the lung or the stomach. The six pulses are wide, big and tight. This condition is caused by kidney energy damage.

C.V.4 *(Guanyuan)*, three hundred times

Avoid taking any herbal formula which is strongly yang in character or produces heat. They are definitely contraindicated for use in this case. If pneumonia shows itself in the six pulses very strong and tight it means that the kidney energy is escaping. In pneumonia cases, saving the kidney energy is the most important thing.

7. Edema when the patient is not able to urinate. The patient cannot breathe upon lying down. The main cause is extreme damage to the spleen energy.

Sp.17 *(Shidou)*, two hundred times
C.V.4 *(Guanyuan)*, three hundred times.

8. Very strong, constantly running diarrhea caused by deficiency of the spleen and finally damages the kidney energy. This situation can possibly cause death.

Sp.17 *(Shidou)*, two hundred times
C.V.4 *(Guanyuan)*, two hundred times.

9. Diarrhea caused by poor diet or indigestion. If the colors keep changing for two to three months it is threatening to the patient's life. This diarrhea shows changing colors because the spleen energy is damaged.

Sp.17 *(Shidou)*, three hundred times
C.V.4 *(Guanyuan)*, three hundred times.

10. Strong stomach cramps, vomiting and diarrhea caused by cold energy damage to the stomach. If this patient has cold arms and legs, and the six pulses are all thin, you have to save the yang energy immediately by applying moxa:

C.V.12 *(Zhongwan)*, fifty times
C.V.4 *(Guanyuan)*, three hundred times.

11. Malaria or any type of condition where fever and chills alternate because cold energy stagnates in the internal organs.
If this problem is only caused by a digestive organ condition, the patient will get better within ten to fifteen days. But if the spleen is damaged and energy is lost through the spleen, the patient will loose vital energy and die.

C.V.12 *(Zhongwan)*, one hundred times
Sp.17 *(Shidou)*, one hundred times only on the left side.

12. Jaundice with yellow eyes, one side of the body yellow, red colored urine caused by cold energy damage to the spleen
If the patient eats any cold food or takes cold energy herbs, the condition will turn into black jaundice and it will be fatal. The patients should not have any sexual intercourse; if they do, they will most certainly damage their kidney energy in which case we have to also moxa G.V.4 *(Mingmen)* three hundred times.

Sp.17 *(Shidou)*, one hundred times.

13. Vomiting and loss of appetite due to spleen damage.

Sp.17 *(Shidou)*, three hundred times.

14. Heat arising very strongly causing the patient to loose consciousness and faint.

C.V.12 *(Zhongwan)*, fifty times.

15. The patient has had a stroke and also displays a mental condition indicating that the heart energy is damaged. Very often this patient will also suffer from insomnia.

C.V.15 *(Jiuwei)*, seventy times.

If they have a skin infection at the same time, also moxa St.36 *(Zusanli)* fifty times.

16. Strong pain on the side of the chest and the patient cannot digest.

Sp.17 *(Shidou)*, one hundred times on the left side.

17. Pain on both sides of the chest turning around the heart is usually considered as pain around the diaphragm. It is caused by strong emotional stress accompanied by continuous anxiety attacks. Usually it is accompanied by hypoglycemia or nervous breakdown. If this problem continues for a long time, a blockage usually develops around the diaphragm area. The three organs involved are the liver, spleen and the kidney. These are also the three organs usually involved in anxiety and nervous breakdown.

At first, anger damages the liver, then the liver damages the spleen and the kidney. When these three organs are drained a blockage usually develops around the diaphragm area. It goes across the liver and the spleen, but they usually show more pain on the left side.

This formula tonifies the liver, spleen and kidney directly. The left Sp.17 *(Shidou)* point is for the spleen, and the right is for the liver.

Sp.17 *(Shidou)*, two hundred times.
C.V.4 *(Guanyuan)*, three hundred times.

18. When the lungs and the respiratory system are damaged by eating cold food, drinking cold drinks or taking cold energy herb formulas, the chest will feel bloated, especially around the xyphoid process. If the patient vomits, they only vomit gastric acid. They feel tired and they always sigh or yawn. Their muscles are tired and their tongue has a white coating. Basically when their respiratory condition is caused by excessive cold energy, you should moxa:

Lu.1 *(Zhongfu)*, two hundred times.

This is an unusual moxibustion formula because the lung is usually damaged by the heat and Lu.1 *(Zhongfu)* is the sedation point. But in this case the lung is damaged by the cold and the way you know it is that their pulse will be tight and sinking. It will look almost normal but you have to notice its sinking aspect. In a typical case of lung congestion, the lung's pulse, no matter how deep or high, feels sandy. There are small vibrations that feel like sand; if they are slight it is a viral damage, if they are high it is bacterial damage. This sensation of sandiness shows that the heat is damaging the lung.

But in the case where this moxibustion formula is applicable, the pulse will be tight and deep. They might also show mucous and tightness around the diaphragm. They may not have any fever or chills. The patient feels better when they breathe in hot air. In this case, you have to give heat to the lungs by moxibustion at Lu.1 *(Zhongfu)*.

We use only Lu.1 *(Zhongfu)* since the cold condition originated in the stomach. Here we are dealing with a *Shang Han* respiratory condition. If we eat cold food in the summer it can damage the spleen or the kidney; it does not have to damage the lung necessarily. But here we *are* talking about a respiratory condition. Cold might not damage the spleen because it always has a bit of heat in it, so the cold bypasses it and goes to the lungs. When cold energy stagnates in the metal element and there is no communication with the earth, the yang part of the spleen can push it out toward the metal. When vomiting gastric acid occurs in this case it is the yang energy from the stomach moving upward. So the yang energy goes towards the metal, but since the metal energy is isolated, it just pushes it out.

19. For asthma or chronic cough condition when chronic coughing is caused by cold energy stagnation in the lung meridian or the lung:

C.V.22 *(Tiantu)*, fifty times.

20. For chronic cough, moxa:

U.B.17 *(Geshu)*, *Koushu* or the mouth *Shu* points.

21. If you suspect cold energy has damaged the respiratory system and might cause pneumonia in the future, or, if the patient is over forty years old and had a coughing problem for a long time:

C.V.4 *(Guanyuan)*, three hundred times.

22. When a patient lies down in a damp and windy area and picks up a perverse energy which enters into the organs and causes hemiplegia. Another condition is when the two eyeballs move separately and both hands are very stiff.

These conditions describe false *Zhong Feng*. Moxa the five yin organ *Shu* points in the following order. If the "A" formula works, then the course of treatment has been completed; if it does not work, then go on to the next treatment, etc.

A. U.B.13 *(Feishu)*, fifty times

B. U.B.13 *(Feishu)*
U.B.15 *(Xinshu)*
Moxa each fifty times.

C. U.B.18 *(Ganshu)*
U.B.23 *(Shenshu)*
Moxa each fifty times.

D.
U.B.13 *(Feishu)*
U.B.15 *(Xinshu)*
U.B.18 *(Ganshu)*
U.B.20 *(Pishu)*
U.B.23 *(Shenshu)*
Moxa each fifty times.

23. In summer, when the patient exhibits dry heat because of damage to the spleen, stomach, and kidney caused by excessive consumption of cold food:

Sp.17 *(Shidou)*, two hundred times

24. If a patient shows pain in the middle of the chest or around the diaphragm, and if the pain is very strong:

Sp.17 *(Shidou)*, fifty times on the left side.

This is basically a continuation of case number 23. If anybody gives cold herbs to this patient, it will kill him. Through excessive consumption of cold food and liquids, the patient develops a blockage in the middle warmer; so there is no communication with the upper warmer and dry heat symptoms might show. But some practitioners might see that they are exhibiting a lot of cramps and dry vomiting where nothing comes out and think that by giving the patient cold herbs and causing vomiting he might save the condition by connecting the two warmers. This will kill the patient by cutting all the connections between the upper, lower and middle warmers. Once that happens they will die within a few hours; even moxa is helpless in that case. The only thing that might save the patient is intravenous glucose or bleeding the back *Shu* points.

25. For paralysis, the old Taoist method has been traditionally recommended:

G.V.20 *(Baihui)*, thirty times
G.B.21 *(Jianjing)*, fifty times
L.I.11 *(Quchi)*, fifty times
St.36 *(Zusanli)*, fifty times.

This combination of points is also a very popular acupuncture formula. It can be a good method, but Bian Que believes that it is not the most suitable one. According to him, the best way to treat paralysis is by moxibustion on C.V.4 *(Guanyuan)* five hundred times.

From my own clinical experience, if the paralysis is mild and the patient has little or no feeling yet can still move with difficulty, the Taoist method does work nicely. If they cannot move at all and are almost in a coma, the Bian Que's method is more appropriate.

The method utilizing C.V.4 *(Guanyuan)* does not always work. If the stroke happens because of a nerve or kidney problem it is an ideal form of treatment, but if it is caused by diabetes, spleen or heat going up, this formula would not work as well.

But it is still good for increasing vital energy, especially when they are loosing it. This method will strengthen the patient.

The first method utilizes a selection of points which is very important for paralysis. If the case shows that moxa is preferred over needling, these points will work better then singular application of C.V.4 *(Guanyuan)*.

26. If a paralysis patient looses speech because the kidney and lung energies are damaged:

C.V.4 *(Guanyuan)*, five hundred times.

27. Intestinal hemorrhage, that does not stop. Usually it is caused by cold energy from food that damages the large intestine. In this case moxa directly on the umbilicus, right in the middle.

C.V.8 *(Shenque)*, thirty times.

28. Physical exhaustion in younger patients, and older patients with constipation due to general debility or weakness caused by other an illness. When they are unable to take any tonification herbs, C.V.8 *(Shenque)* is good for intestinal problems while C.V.4 *(Guanyuan)* is better for intestinal problems related to kidney energy.

C.V.8 *(Shenque)*, one hundred times.

29. Blood in the urine due to damage of the bladder or kidney. Usually it is because of kidney energy damage due to excessive sex:

C.V.4 *(Guanyuan)*, two hundred times.

30. Bladder infection or mild gonorrhea caused by heat damaging the kidney water energy. This clearly demonstrates the fact that C.V.4 *(Guanyuan)* does not promote heat from moxibustion but another form of energy which, in this case, increases the kidney water energy.

C.V.4 *(Guanyuan)*, three hundred times.

31. Diabetes in patients who are very thirsty and drinking two to three liters of water everyday. This occurs because their heart and kidney are damaged by the heat. It can also happen due to cold energy from food damaging the lung and the kidney. We use C.V.6 *(Qihai)* in the spring because the energy is growing and the kidney energy is at its peak. So we can work in the higher part of the body. In this case even if we are using C.V.6 *(Qihai)*, we are still tonifying C.V.4 *(Guanyuan)*.

C.V.4 *(Guanyuan)* or C.V.6 *(Qihai)*, one hundred times.

32. Diabetes showing great appetite and very weak legs and arms. This is because spleen, kidney, and stomach are very deficient. In this case we are tonifying the kidney so it can tonify the other organs.

C.V.4 *(Guanyuan)*, five hundred times.

33. The lower back and legs are very stiff. The patient cannot flex them or walk. This is caused by loss of kidney energy through excessive sexual activity or illness. This condition can damage the bones in the back.

C.V.4 *(Guanyuan)*, five hundred times.

34. The patient is unconscious and cannot swallow food. Or, if the patient can move, he moves around in a haze or insensible. If this condition is caused by a nervous breakdown, anxiety or depression:

C.V.14 *(Juque)*, fifty times.

35. Spleen damage that shows black or yellowish color on the face and loss of appetite.

Sp.17 *(Shidou)*, fifty times on the left side.

If this patient has a very pale complexion there is additionally kidney damage, therefore also moxa C.V.4 *(Guanyuan)* two hundred times.

36. If wind *(feng)* goes in through the ear and the patient shows facial palsy (Bell's Palsy).

St.4 *(Dicang)* twenty-seven or fifty times.

37. If both ears show dryness and grayish or black color it is an indication of kidney energy damage.

C.V.4 *(Guanyuan)*, five hundred times.

38. For patients over 40 years old with a dry mouth and tongue, there is no salivation. This is because the kidney energy is low and no longer generating adequate water energy

C.V.4 *(Guanyuan)*, three hundred times.

39. If a patient over forty years old has strong pain in the lower back and the sacrum, it is usually because the kidney energy is damaged and wind penetrates that area. If we give any metal-hot type of herbal formula to this patient in attempting to eliminate that wind, the condition may worsen.

C.V.4 *(Guanyuan)*, three hundred times.

40. When there is inflammation of the skin in the groin area because kidney energy is attacked by perverse wind energy

penetrating to the bone, the patient's condition may develop into a bone disease.

C.V.4 *(Guanyuan)*, two hundred times.

41. For patients over sixty years old whose intestines are loose and their urination shows no strength. This can lead to either constipation or diarrhea. Their yang energy is very low which results in their inability to control their elimination.

C.V.8 *(Shenque)*, three hundred times.

42. For older patients whose breathing is short and shallow. Their kidney energy is not returning from the lung to the kidney. The contact between lung and kidney is cut, especially from top to bottom. In this case such patients may hyperventilate.

C.V.4 *(Guanyuan)*, two hundred times.

43. For older patients who have no control over the rectal muscles because their spleen and kidney energy are exhausted. In this case they cannot control excretion and it comes out all the time.

Sp.17 *(Shidou)*, two hundred times on the left side,
C.V.4 *(Guanyuan)*, two hundred times.

44. For cataract. When the patient's eyesight is failing and the cataract is very darkly pigmented. This is because the spleen and kidney energy are very depleted.

C.V.4 *(Guanyuan)*, three hundred times.

45. Serious and very deep skin infection on the scalp. It is usually due to liver damage caused by depression and worry, or poisonous food. Liver diseases may attack the scalp because the liver receives its yang heat poison through the gall bladder meridian.

Moxa thirty-seven times right on top of the pus itself.

This formula is a bit radical. Often when there is deep skin infection you can moxa right on top and the moxa will actually sedate the infection. It is like drying up the heat in the liquid form. If the infection is deep on the buttocks or thigh this method will also work; you can moxa about fifty times without any problem. This method works for the scalp, but make sure that you use enough moxa cones to effectively sedate the infection.

46. Tetanus when the jaws are getting tight and the cervical and the upper thoracic vertebrae are also becoming tight. This formula works for tetanus only when the jaws and vertebrae are both tightening.

C.V.4 *(Guanyuan)*, one hundred times.

47. Lower backache with cold and damp energy.

G.V.2 *(Yaoshu)*, fifty times.

48. When the patient has painful knees or thighs and is unable to walk and a few points, usually on top of the kneecap or the lateral surface of the thighs, are especially painful.

Pick out *Ahshi* or painful points and moxa them thirty times.

49. Weak, stiff, and swollen leg or Beriberi.

Kd.1 *(Yongquan)*, fifty times.

50. Skin dryness in adults and children including psoriasis. When the skin forms dry patches and there is no sweat coming out of the pores.

Moxibustion three *cuns* away from the center of the dry patch.

Determine the meridian's direction and choose two points -- one above and one below. If the meridian line is not clear, pick out four points, one on each side. Moxa each point three times. If the points secrete yellow fluid, which is usually lymph, then it is a sign of healing. Continue this treatment until the fluid comes out.

INDEX

D

M

Ma Wang Tui, v, vi
Malaria, 27, 37, 48
Menopause, 27
Menstrual Disorders, 27
Mental condition, 37, 49
Methods of treatment, 2
Middle warmer, 42, 52, 53
Migraine, 17, 43
Ming Dynasty, vi
Mingguan, 41
Miscarriage, 21
Mouth, 14
Moxibustion, v
Myopia, 14

N, O

Nei Jing, ix
Nerve, 28, 53
Nervous breakdown, 49, 55
Neuralgia, 38
Night blindness, 14
Nose, 14, 15
Numbness, 23
Nutrition, 2
Odor, 11
Osteoporosis, 28, 36

P, Q, R

Pain, ix, 17, 22, 23, 24, 25, 32, 38, 43, 49, 52, 56
Painful after delivery, 42
Painful knees, 58
Painful points, 58
Painful swelling, 42
Paralysis, 16, 28, 31, 34, 36, 42, 45, 53, 54
Pathogenic factors, 46
Pc.8 *(Laogong)*, 12
Periods, 36
Pharmacology, vi
Physical therapy, 2
Pneumonia, 28, 47, 51
Polyps, 15
Prevention of Disease, 26
Psoriasis, 31, 59
Pulses, viii, 3, 7, 11, 30, 34, 35, 45, 46, 47, 48, 50
Pus, 23, 30, 46, 58
Qing Dynasties, vi
Respiratory condition, 50
Respiratory system, 50, 51

S

S.I.5 *(Yanggu)*, 17
S.I.10 *(Naoshu)*, 23
S.I.19 *(Tinggong)*, 14
Sacrum, 24, 25, 56
Salt, 5
Scarring, vii
Sciatica, 24, 29
Sedation, 3, 5, 6
Seizures, 29, 36, 42
Sex drive, 21
Sexual activity, 54, 55
Sexual deficiency, 20, 21

THE HEART & ESSENCE Of Dan-xi's Methods of Treatment by Zhu Dan-xi, trans. by Yang Shou-zhong. ISBN 0-936185-50-3, $24.95

HOW TO WRITE A TCM HERBAL FORMULA A Logical Methodology for the Formulation & Administration of Chinese Herbal Medicine in Decoction, by Bob Flaws, ISBN 0-936185-49-X, $10.95

FULFILLING THE ESSENCE: A Handbook of Traditional & Contemporary Chinese Treatments for Female Infertility by Bob Flaws. ISBN 0-936185-48-1, $19.95

STATEMENTS OF FACT IN TRADITIONAL CHINESE MEDICINE by Bob Flaws. ISBN 0-936185-52-X, $10.95

IMPERIAL SECRETS OF HEALTH & LONGEVITY by Bob Flaws, ISBN 0-936185-51-1, $9.95

THE MEDICAL I CHING: Oracle of the Healer Within by Miki Shima, OMD, ISBN 0-936185-38-4, $19.95

THE SYSTEMATIC CLASSIC OF ACUPUNCTURE /MOXIBUSTION by Huang-fu Mi, trans. by Yang Shou-zhong and Charles Chace, ISBN 0-936185-29-5, hardback edition, $79.95

CHINESE PEDIATRIC MASSAGE THERAPY A Parent's & Practitioner's Guide to the Treatment and Prevention of Childhood Disease, by Fan Ya-li. ISBN 0-936185-54-6, $12.95

RECENT TCM RESEARCH FROM CHINA trans. by Bob Flaws & Charles Chace. ISBN 0-936185-56-2, $18.95

PMS: Its Cause, Diagnosis & Treatment According to Traditional Chinese Medicine by Bob Flaws ISBN 0-936185-22-8 $16.95

EXTRA TREATISES BASED ON INVESTIGATION & INQUIRY: A Translation of Zhu Dan-xi's Ge Zhi Yu Lun, trans. by Yang Shou-zhong & Duan Wu-jin, ISBN 0-936185-53-8, $15.95

THE DIVINELY
RESPONDING CLASSIC: A
Translation of the *Shen Ying
Jing* by Yang Shou-zhong and
Liu Feng-ting, ISBN 0-936185-
55-4, $18.95

A NEW AMERICAN
ACUPUNCTURE:
Acupuncture Osteopathy, by Mark
Seem, ISBN 0-936185-44-9,
$19.95

SCATOLOGY & THE
GATE OF LIFE: The Role
of the Large Intestine in
Immunity, An Integrated
Chinese-Western Approach
by Bob Flaws ISBN 0-936185-20-
1 $14.95

MENOPAUSE, A Second
Spring: Making A Smooth
Transition with Traditional
Chinese Medicine by Honora
Lee Wolfe ISBN 0-936185-18-X
$14.95

MIGRAINES &
TRADITIONAL CHINESE
MEDICINE: A Layperson's
Guide by Bob Flaws ISBN 0-
936185-15-5 $11.95

STICKING TO THE
POINT: A Rational
Methodology for the Step by
Step Administration of an
Acupuncture Treatment by
Bob Flaws ISBN 0-936185-17-1
$16.95

ENDOMETRIOSIS &
INFERTILITY AND
TRADITIONAL CHINESE
MEDICINE: A Laywoman's
Guide by Bob Flaws ISBN 0-
936185-14-7 $9.95

THE BREAST
CONNECTION: A
Laywoman's Guide to the
Treatment of Breast Disease
by Chinese Medicine
by Honora Lee Wolfe ISBN 0-
936185-61-9 $9.95

NINE OUNCES: A Nine Part
Program For The Prevention
of AIDS in HIV Positive
Persons by Bob Flaws ISBN 0-
936185-12-0 $9.95

THE TREATMENT OF
CANCER BY
INTEGRATED
CHINESE-WESTERN
MEDICINE by Zhang Dai-
zhao, trans. by Zhang Ting-liang
ISBN 0-936185-11-2 $18.95

A HANDBOOK OF
TRADITIONAL CHINESE
DERMATOLOGY by Liang
Jian-hui, trans. by Zhang Ting-
liang & Bob Flaws, ISBN 0-
936185-07-4 $15.95

A HANDBOOK OF
TRADITIONAL CHINESE
GYNECOLOGY by Zhejiang
College of TCM, trans. by Zhang
Ting-liang, ISBN 0-936185-06-6
(2nd edit.) $21.95

PRINCE WEN HUI'S
COOK: Chinese Dietary
Therapy by Bob Flaws &
Honora Lee Wolfe, ISBN 0-
912111-05-4, $12.95 (Published by
Paradigm Press, Brookline, MA)

THE DAO OF
INCREASING LONGEVITY
AND CONSERVING ONE'S
LIFE by Anna Lin & Bob Flaws,
ISBN 0-936185-24-4 $16.95

FIRE IN THE VALLEY:
The TCM Diagnosis and
Treatment of Vaginal
Diseases by Bob Flaws
ISBN 0-936185-25-2 $16.95

HIGHLIGHTS OF
ANCIENT ACUPUNCTURE
PRESCRIPTIONS trans. by
Honora Lee Wolfe & Rose
Crescenz ISBN 0-936185-23-6
$14.95

ARISAL OF THE CLEAR:
A Simple Guide to Healthy
Eating According to
Traditional Chinese Medicine
by Bob Flaws, ISBN #-936185-
27-9 $8.95

PEDIATRIC BRONCHITIS:
ITS CAUSE, DIAGNOSIS &
TREATMENT
ACCORDING TO
TRADITIONAL CHINESE
MEDICINE trans. by Gao Yu-li
and Bob Flaws, ISBN 0-936185-
26-0 $15.95

AIDS & ITS TREATMENT
ACCORDING TO
TRADITIONAL CHINESE
MEDICINE by Huang Bing-
shan, trans. by Fu-Di & Bob
Flaws, ISBN 0-936185-28-7
$24.95

ACUTE ABDOMINAL
SYNDROMES: Their
Diagnosis & Treatment by
Combined Chinese-Western
Medicine by Alon Marcus, ISBN
0-936185-31-7 $16.95

MY SISTER, THE MOON:
The Diagnosis & Treatment
of Menstrual Diseases by
Traditional Chinese Medicine
by Bob Flaws, ISBN 0-936185-
34-1, $24.95

FU QING-ZHU'S
GYNECOLOGY trans. by
Yang Shou-zhong and Liu Da-
wei, ISBN 0-936185-35-X,
$21.95

FLESHING OUT THE
BONES: The Importance of
Case Histories in Chinese
Medicine by Charles Chace.
ISBN 0-936185-30-9, $18.95

CLASSICAL
MOXIBUSTION SKILLS
IN CONTEMPORARY
CLINICAL PRACTICE by
Sung Baek, ISBN 0-936185-16-3
$10.95

MASTER TONG'S
ACUPUNCTURE: An
Ancient Lineage for Modern
Practice, trans. and commentary
by Miriam Lee, OMD, ISBN 0-
936185-37-6, $19.95

A HANDBOOK OF TCM
UROLOGY & MALE
SEXUAL DYSFUNCTION by
Anna Lin, OMD, ISBN 0-936185-
36-8, $16.95

Li Dong-yuan's TREATISE
ON THE SPLEEN &
STOMACH, A Translation
of the *Pi Wei Lun* by Yang
Shou-zhong & Li Jian-yong, ISBN
0-936185-41-4, $21.95

PATH OF PREGNANCY,
VOL. I, Gestational
Disorders by Bob Flaws, ISBN
0-936185-39-2, $16.95

PATH OF PREGNANCY,
VOL. II, Postpartum
Diseases by Bob Flaws, ISBN
0-936185-42-2, $18.95

How to Have a HEALTHY
PREGNANCY, HEALTHY
BIRTH with Traditional
Chinese Medicine by Honora Lee
Wolfe, ISBN 0-936185-40-6,
$9.95

MASTER HUA'S CLASSIC
OF THE CENTRAL
VISCERA by Hua Tuo,
translated by Yang Shou-zhong,
ISBN 0-936185-43-0, $21.95

SEVENTY ESSENTIAL
TCM FORMULAS FOR
BEGINNERS by Bob Flaws,
ISBN 0-936185-59-7, $19.95